CHAIR YOGA FOR SENIORS

Enhance Flexibility and Strength

Johnson Myers

Disclaimer

This book, "Chair Yoga for Seniors," is intended to provide general information about yoga poses and exercises that can be done with a chair as a prop, and is designed to help seniors maintain their health and wellbeing.

It is important to note that yoga, like any physical activity, carries inherent risks. While the poses and exercises in this book are generally safe, they may not be appropriate for everyone, particularly those with certain health conditions or injuries.

Readers are strongly advised to consult with their physician before beginning any new exercise program, especially if they have any concerns about their health or physical abilities.

Table of Contents

Introduction

As we age, it becomes increasingly important to prioritize our physical and mental health. For seniors, staying active and maintaining mobility can be challenging. However, one practice that has been shown to have numerous benefits for seniors is chair yoga.

Chair yoga is a gentle form of yoga that is adapted for those who have mobility or balance issues. It involves performing yoga poses while sitting on a chair or using a chair for support. This makes it a perfect fit for seniors who may struggle with traditional yoga practices.

One of the main benefits of chair yoga is improved flexibility, which can help seniors move more freely and with less pain. Chair yoga also helps to build strength and balance, reducing the risk of falls and injuries. In addition, chair yoga is a low-impact form of exercise that can help manage joint pain and reduce stress.

One inspiring story of the benefits of chair yoga is that of a senior named Maya. Maya had suffered from arthritis and chronic pain for years, which made it difficult for her to move around and participate in physical activity. However, after attending a chair yoga class, she found that she was able to move more freely and with less pain. As she continued to practice chair yoga, she noticed significant improvements in her overall physical and mental well-being.

Maya's experience is not unique. Many seniors have found that chair yoga has helped them maintain their health and independence as they age. In fact, a study conducted by the University of California, Los Angeles found that seniors who practiced chair yoga had improved physical and mental health outcomes compared to those who did not practice yoga.

One of the reasons chair yoga is so effective for seniors is that it can be easily modified to fit different abilities. For example, those with limited mobility can perform seated poses that help to stretch and strengthen their muscles. Those who are more mobile can incorporate standing poses with the support of a chair.

In addition to physical benefits, chair yoga also has numerous mental health benefits for seniors. Chair yoga helps to reduce stress and anxiety, improve mental clarity and focus, and enhance overall well-being. For seniors who may be experiencing feelings of loneliness or isolation, attending a chair yoga class can also be a great way to socialize and connect with others.

If you are a senior over 60 and are interested in trying chair yoga, there are a few things to keep in mind. First, it is important to set up your practice space in a safe and comfortable manner. You will also want to wear comfortable clothing and have any necessary equipment, such as a chair and yoga blocks, nearby.

It is also important to practice chair yoga with safety in mind. Seniors should be careful not to overexert themselves or push themselves beyond their limits. It is recommended to start slowly and gradually increase the intensity and duration of your practice over time.

Chair yoga is a wonderful practice for seniors over 60 who want to maintain their physical and mental health. Maya's story is just one example of how chair yoga can be a life-changing practice for seniors. With consistent practice, you may find that chair yoga helps you maintain your health and independence well into your golden years.

Chapter One

Introduction to Yoga

Yoga has a 4,000-year history that begins in ancient India. As most of yoga's early history was handed down orally, its roots are relatively obscure. Yet it's said that yoga was first created as a means of achieving enlightenment.

The Rigveda, a body of old Hindu writings, which dates back to roughly 1500 BCE, has the oldest reference of yoga. The Rigveda makes reference to a number of techniques that are still essential to modern yoga practice, such as breathing exercises, meditation, and the recitation of mantras.

Yoga changed and got more organized over time. In 400 CE, Patanjali composed his collection of yoga aphorisms, known as the Yoga Sutras. The eight limbs of yoga, which consist of meditation, breathing exercises, and physical postures (asanas), are described in these sutras (dhyana).

Throughout the ages, yoga continued to grow, with several schools of yoga emerging in India. Tirumalai Krishnamacharya, who lived from 1888 to 1989, was one of the most significant individuals in the history of yoga. Due to the fact that he trained a number of well-known yoga instructors who later propagated the discipline across Europe and the United States, Krishnamacharya is sometimes credited with introducing yoga to the West.

Yoga started to become more well-liked in the West in the 20th century. Many Americans developed an interest in yoga throughout the 1960s and 1970s as a result of a larger cultural trend toward Eastern spirituality and alternative lifestyles. Yoga became a well-liked method of exercise and stress alleviation as yoga studios spread throughout the nation.

Currently, millions of people all around the globe practice yoga. From sportsmen and celebrities to spiritual searchers and those searching for a method to manage stress and enhance their general health and well-being, it has been embraced by a diverse group of people. While yoga has evolved and adapted to meet the demands of contemporary practitioners, its origins in ancient India continue to be an important element of its past and present.

The part of yoga that Westerners are most familiar with are the physical positions, or asanas. They are designed to improve range of motion, flexibility, strength, and balance. Each asana is intended to focus on a different area of the body, and consistent practice may result in an improvement in general health and wellbeing.

Pranayama, or breathing exercises, are a crucial component of yoga. Exercises in pranayama may soothe anxiety and tension while increasing oxygenation of the body's tissues and calming the mind. In order to develop the practice, they often go hand in hand with the physical postures and include conscious control of the breath.

Another crucial component of yoga is meditation, it entails concentrating the attention on a certain thing or concept, which may ease tension, enhance mental clarity, and foster a feeling of inner serenity. To establish a whole mind-body practice, meditation is often done with asanas and pranayama.

Yoga contains moral guidelines known as the yamas and niyamas in addition to these physical exercises. The yamas are moral principles for relating to the world, and they encompass ideas like non-violence, honesty, and non-attachment. The niyamas are a set of personal ethical principles that encompass ideas like self-control, contentment, and introspection.

Yoga comes in a wide variety of forms, each with its own special emphasis and methodology. Among the most well-liked looks are:

Hatha yoga is a moderate, beginner-friendly form of exercise that emphasizes fundamental poses and breathing techniques.

Vinyasa yoga is a dynamic, flow-based technique that combines movement and breathing.

Ashtanga yoga is a strenuous, traditional exercise that calls for a predetermined sequence of poses.

Bikram yoga is an exercise regimen that calls for doing a predetermined series of poses in a warm environment.

Iyengar yoga is a kind of exercise that places a strong emphasis on posture alignment and accuracy, often using straps and blocks as supports.

Both the mind and the body may gain greatly from yoga. It may enhance balance, flexibility, and strength as well as lower tension and anxiety and boost overall health and wellbeing. Through consistent practice, yoga may foster inner tranquility and a stronger feeling of connectedness to oneself and the world around one.

Introduction to Chair Yoga

When a chair is used to support and adjust standard yoga positions in a kind of yoga, it is known as "chair yoga." The chair may give stability for balance, assistance for those with restricted mobility, and a safe method to do yoga postures that can be difficult or impossible to do on the floor. Anybody may do chair yoga, including elderly, those with impairments or injuries, as well as those who just want a more gentle form of yoga. While it is often taught while sitting, it may also include standing or utilizing a chair as a prop for certain stretches and postures.

How Seniors Can Do Chair Yoga

By using a chair to support and modify classic yoga positions, chair yoga is a modified style of yoga designed for seniors. For seniors, chair yoga may be modified in a number of ways:

Modifications to the Chair

The chair is utilized as a prop to support the body and assist elders in doing yoga postures safely and comfortably. For instance, twists may be performed while holding onto the back of the chair, and sitting forward folds can be performed with the feet on the floor or on blocks.

Gentle Movements

Chair yoga focuses on easy-to-do postures and stretches that assist enhance flexibility, mobility, and strength. The exercises are performed carefully and slowly, and the teacher may suggest adjustments to assist students with varying degrees of mobility.

Both sitting and standing positions are possible while practicing chair yoga. Standing versions that utilize the chair as support are also possible. Seniors may do standing leg lifts with one hand on the chair for assistance or standing forward folds with both hands on the chair.

Breath Work and Meditation

To assist seniors, relax, relieve tension, and enhance mental clarity, chair yoga often incorporates breath work exercises and meditation methods. These exercises may be performed either while sitting in the chair or while standing and using the chair as a prop.

Chair yoga is modified for seniors with an emphasis on safety, incorporating changes and adaptations that assist lower the chance of injury. In addition to encouraging elders to listen to their bodies and adjust postures as necessary, the teacher may provide advice on good alignment and posture.

Seniors of all mobility and fitness levels may use chair yoga as a gentle and convenient form of exercise. Seniors may safely and easily practice yoga and benefit from its many physical and mental health advantages by using a chair for support and adjustment.

Chapter Two

Basic Guidelines for Chair Yoga Practice for Seniors over 60

For seniors over 60 who desire to practice chair yoga, here are some general rules:

Communicate with Your Health Facilitator

Before beginning any new workout program, it's crucial to speak with your healthcare practitioner to be sure it's safe for you to do so.

Locate a Knowledgeable Teacher

Seek for a certified yoga teacher with knowledge in instructing elders in chair yoga. They may help you with the positions and make sure you're doing them correctly and securely.

Wear Comfortable Clothing

Dress comfortably and loosely so that you may move about without being constrained.

Use a Strong Chair

Choose for a robust chair that is not too high or low and does not have wheels. A backrest and stability are required for the chair.

Take Note of Your Body and Strength

Practice at a rate that seems comfortable to you by paying attention to your body. Modify or skip a position if it hurts or seems too tough.

Take Note of Your Breathing

Breathing is a key component of yoga, so pay attention to it. Throughout each posture, pay attention to inhaling slowly and deeply and expelling completely.

Stay Hydrated

Keep hydrated by drinking plenty of water before, during, and after your practice.

Take Breaks as Necessary

If you feel the need to relax or take a break, do so. Do not do more than you can handle.

Be Dependable

When it comes to reaping the advantages of yoga, consistency is essential. Even for a little time each day, try to routinely engage in chair yoga.

Seniors over 60 may practice chair yoga safely and successfully while reaping its numerous advantages by adhering to these fundamental rules.

Yoga Equipment and Tools

To guarantee a secure and pleasant practice, it's crucial to utilize the necessary tools and dress comfortably and appropriately for chair yoga. Here are some recommendations for attire and tools for practicing chair yoga:

Clothing

- Dress comfortably and with ease of mobility in mind. Pick lightweight, breathable apparel that won't impede your mobility.
- While practicing, stay away from loose or baggy clothes that might snag on the chair or your body.
- To adapt to temperature variations during practice, dress in layers.
- Avoid putting on jewelry or accessories that might hurt you or interfere with your practice.

Equipment

- Practice of chair yoga requires a solid chair with a backrest. Verify that the chair is sturdy and free of wheels.

- A rug or yoga mat with a non-slip surface may provide support and stop slippage.
- Blocks, blankets, and straps are examples of props that may be used to alter and improve postures.
- It's crucial to bring a water bottle to practice in order to keep hydrated.

Prioritize comfort and safety while selecting yoga tools and attires for chair practice. Avoid wearing or using anything during practice that might make you uncomfortable or hurt yourself.

Adaptations and Variations for Various Abilities

Seniors of all levels of mobility and fitness may benefit from chair yoga since it is a flexible type of yoga that can be tweaked and customized to meet their requirements. Here are several chair yoga adaptations and variants for various skill levels:

Variations for Sitting

Several classic yoga positions may be adapted for a sitting position. For instance, forward folds and twists performed when sitting are mild variations of those performed while standing.

Employ Props

You may alter positions and make them more accessible by using items like blankets, blocks, and straps. For instance, in sitting forward folds, blocks may be utilized to bring the floor closer to the body.

Chair Support

In several positions, a chair may be utilized as a support. For instance, gripping onto the chair's sides to maintain balance when standing or utilizing the chair's back for support.

Seniors might benefit from mild activities like wrist circles, neck stretches, and shoulder rolls. These exercises may increase flexibility and mobility.

Breathing Techniques

To ease tension and encourage relaxation, chair yoga practices may include breathing techniques. Deep breathing and alternating nostril breathing are two examples.

Visualization

Seniors may employ visualizations to relax and concentrate while practicing. For instance, visualizing a serene setting, such a beach or mountain, may aid in promoting relaxation.

Weighted Chair Yoga

Doing chair yoga with little weights may assist older citizens increase their strength and enhance their bone density. But before incorporating weights into their routine, seniors should speak with their doctor.

Chapter Three

Chair Yoga Poses for Seniors over 60

Breathing Techniques

Yoga practice is not complete without pranayama, often known as breathing exercises. These include regulating the breath in certain ways to enhance both physical and mental wellbeing. Yoga offers a variety of breathing exercises that may be used to get various results.

Diaphragmatic Breathing

This is sometimes referred to as belly breathing, includes taking slow, deep breaths into the diaphragm to soothe tension, lessen stress, and expand the lung capacity. Sit comfortably with your hands on your tummy to try this technique. Inhale gently via your nose, allowing air to fill your belly. Gently tense your abdominal muscles while you breathe out through your lips to push the air out.

Ujjayi Breathing

In order to produce a "hissing" sound, this method requires inhaling via the nose while tightening the back of the throat. Many yoga programs employ ujjayi breathing to encourage calmness and concentration as well as to control the breath during difficult positions. To use this method, take a deep breath in via your nose, then exhale while tightening the back of your throat.

Alternate Nostril Breathing

This technique involves alternating the breath between the left and right nostrils to balance the body's energy and calm the mind. To practice this technique, sit comfortably with your left hand resting on your left knee and your right hand in front of your face. Using your right thumb, close your right nostril and inhale deeply through your left nostril. Then, using your right ring finger, close your left nostril and exhale through your right nostril. Repeat the process, inhaling through your right nostril and exhaling through your left nostril.

Kapalabhati Breathing

To improve energy, stimulate the digestive system, and eliminate toxins, this method includes quick, strong exhalations via the nose. Sit comfortably with your hands on your tummy to try this technique. Deeply inhale through your nose, forcing your breath out through your nose while tightening your abdominal muscles. Passively inhale, then violently expel once more. Repeat a number of times.

Deep Breathing

Sit upright in your chair with your feet firm on the ground and take a deep breath. Close your eyes and take a deep breath in to fill your lungs with air. After a brief period of holding your breath, carefully let all the air out of your lungs via your mouth. For many breaths, go through this procedure again while concentrating on how your body feels as the breath enters and exits.

Abdominal Breathing

Put your hands on your tummy and breathe deeply through your nose to practice abdominal breathing. Let your tummy to expand and fill with oxygen as you inhale. Exhale gradually through your lips, allowing your tummy to relax as you do so. Continue doing this for a few breaths, noticing how your tummy rises and falls with each inhalation and exhalation.

Ocean Breath

Sit up straight in your chair and take a deep breath of the ocean. Inhale deeply with your nose, then let the air out through your lips while uttering the word "haaa." For many breaths, repeat this procedure, concentrating on the sound of the breath and the feeling of the air entering and leaving your body.

Yoga breathing exercises may have a significant impact on the body and psyche. You may increase your lung capacity, lessen tension and anxiety, improve your mental clarity and attention, and feel better overall by adding these strategies into your yoga practice. To reap the full benefits of these practices, it is advised to frequently put them into practice.

Warm-up poses

For seniors to keep active and healthy, try chair yoga. Warming up correctly is crucial before starting any physical activity in order to avoid injuries and get the body ready to move. In order to prepare seniors for their chair yoga practice, do these warm-up postures in a chair:

Rolls of the Neck

- Sit up straight on the chair, flat on the floor.

- Roll the head to the right, bringing the right ear to the right shoulder, and gently lower the chin into the chest.

- Hold for a little while, then rotate your head back to the middle and do the opposite on the left side.

Shoulder Rolls

- Roll your shoulders forward in a circular motion while sitting up straight in your chair.

- Repeat 5–10 times, then switch the rolls' axes and do it again.

Side Stretches

- Stretching the sides of the body involves sitting up straight in the chair and raising the right arm upward to the left side of the body.

- After a brief period of holding, drop your arm and repeat on the other side.

Twists While Seated

- Place your feet flat on the ground and sit up straight in the chair.
- Twist your body to the left while utilizing your right hand to further the stretch by placing it on the outside of your left leg.
- Hold for a little while, then let go and repeat on the other side.

Seated Cat-Cow Stretch

- Sit up straight in the chair with the feet flat on the floor to do the seated cat-cow stretch.
- Take a deep breath in and arch your back, moving your shoulders back and your chest forward (cow pose).

- Exhale and round the back, pushing the shoulders forward and the chin into the chest (cat pose).

- Repeat a few times, moving in sync with your breathing.

Forward Folding when Seated

- Place your feet flat on the ground and sit up straight on the chair.

- While you inhale, raise your arms in the air.

- Fold forward while exhaling, bringing the hands to the feet.

- Hold for a little while, then raise yourself back up to a sitting posture gradually.

Seniors who practice chair yoga may warm up their bodies, improve circulation, and lessen bodily stiffness and pain.

Seated poses

Seniors may practice yoga safely and easily by doing postures while seated. Seniors who may have restricted mobility or trouble standing up and down from the floor might benefit greatly from chair yoga. Seniors may do the following sitting yoga positions in a chair:

Mountain Position when Seated

- Place your feet flat on the ground and sit up straight in the chair.
- When you stretch your spine and press your feet firmly into the ground, lift your head's crown toward the ceiling.
- Take a few slow, deep breaths while placing the hands over the heart.

Forward Folding when Seated

- Place your feet flat on the ground and sit up straight on the chair.

- While you inhale, raise your arms in the air.

- Fold forward while exhaling, bringing the hands to the feet.

- Hold for a little while, then raise yourself back up to a sitting posture gradually.

Twist while Seated

- Place your feet flat on the ground and sit up straight in the chair.

- Twist your body to the left while utilizing your right hand to further the stretch by placing it on the outside of your left leg.

- Hold for a little while, then let go and repeat on the other side.

Seated Cat Cow stretch

- Sit up straight in the chair with the feet flat on the floor to do the seated cat-cow stretch.

- Take a deep breath in and arch your back, moving your shoulders back and your chest forward (cow pose).

- Exhale and round the back, pushing the shoulders forward and the chin into the chest (cat pose).

- Repeat many repetitions while controlling your breathing.

Seated Pigeon Pose

- Put your feet flat on the ground and adopt the seated pigeon position.

- While maintaining the right foot flexed, cross the right ankle across the left knee.

- To intensify the stretch, gently push the right knee away from the torso.

- Hold for a little while, then let go and repeat on the other side.

Seated Eagle Pose

- Place the feet flat on the floor and sit up straight on the chair.

- Wrap the right foot around the left calf before crossing the right thigh over the left leg.

- Bending the elbows and bringing the palms together, the right arm is brought underneath the left arm.

- Hold for a little while, then let go and repeat on the other side.

These sitting positions for seniors may enhance circulation, promote flexibility, and lessen body stiffness and pain.

Standing poses with Chair Support

Although still enabling seniors to do yoga positions that may enhance balance, flexibility, and strength, standing poses with chair support can provide them more stability and support. Seniors may attempt the following standing positions while supported by a chair:

Mountain Pose

- Standing with your feet hip-width apart and your toes pointed forward, do Chair Tadasana (Mountain Pose).
- Use both hands to support yourself by clinging to the back of a chair.
- When you stretch your spine and press your feet firmly into the ground, lift your head's crown toward the ceiling.
- Release after a few long breaths.

Chair Forward Fold

- Your toes should be directed forward when you stand with your feet hip-width apart.

- Use both hands to support yourself by clinging to the back of a chair.

- While you inhale, raise your arms in the air.

- Fold forward while exhaling, bringing the hands to the feet.

- Hold for a little while, then gently raise yourself back up to standing.

Chair Warrior

- Standing with your feet wide apart, turn your right foot out to the side.

- To support yourself, grasp the back of a chair with your right hand.

- Maintaining alignment with the ankle, bend the right knee.

- Look over the right hand with the left arm extended to the side.

- Hold for a while, then release, and repeat on the other side.

Chair Tree Pose

- Stand in the chair tree position, toes pointing forward and feet hip-width apart.
- Use both hands to support yourself by clinging to the back of a chair.
- Place the right foot's sole on the inner of the left thigh while shifting your weight to your left foot and raising your right foot off the ground.
- Lengthen your spine and press your foot into your thigh.
- Hold for a while, then release, and repeat on the other side.

Chair Triangle Pose

- Standing with your feet wide apart, bend your right foot out to the side.
- To support yourself, grasp the back of a chair with your right hand.

- Bending at the waist, raise the left arm above
  before bringing the left hand up to the right
  ankle.
- Take a look up at the left hand.
- Hold for a while, then release, and repeat on the
  other side.

These standing exercises for seniors may increase their
strength, flexibility, and balance while also adding
more stability and support.

Backbends and Twist

Seniors may benefit from gentle backbends and twists
to increase their flexibility, mobility, and spinal health.
Seniors may practice the following easy twists and
backbends:

Sitting Spinal Twist

- Place your feet flat on the floor and sit up
  straight in the chair.

- Twisting to the right, place the right hand behind the back and the left hand on the right knee.
- Hold for a while, then release, and repeat on the other side.

Sphinx Position

- Lay on the stomach with the forearms on the floor and the elbows beneath the shoulders.
- Lifting the chest off the ground while gently arching the back, press the forearms down.
- Hold for a while, then release.

Cobra Position

- Lay on the stomach with the elbows close to the body and the hands beneath the shoulders.
- Lifting the chest off the floor while keeping the shoulders down and away from the ears requires pressing the hands and feet firmly into the ground.

- Hold for a while, then release.

Seated Forward Bend with a Twist

- Place your feet flat on the ground and sit up straight in the chair.

- While you inhale, raise your arms in the air.

- Fold forward while exhaling, bringing the hands to the feet.

- Then turn to the right, putting the right hand on the chair's back and the left hand on the right knee.

- Hold for a while, then release, and repeat on the other side.

Bridge Pose

- Lay on your back in the bridge position with your knees bent and your feet flat on the ground.

- By squeezing the feet and arms firmly into the ground, raise the hips off the ground.
- Hold for a while, then release.

Seniors may benefit from these easy backbends and twists because they build flexibility, boost blood flow, and lessen body stiffness and pain.

Forward Folds and Hip Openers

Seniors who practice hip openers and forward folds may increase their flexibility, mobility, and circulation while easing stress and pain in their hips and lower back. Seniors may practice the following hip openers and forward folds:

Butterfly Posture when Seated

- Place your feet flat on the ground and sit up straight in the chair.
- The knees should be left to fall out to the sides while you bring the soles of your feet together.

- Gently push the knees toward the floor while holding onto the feet or ankles with your hands.

- Hold for a little while, then release.

Forward Bend while Seated

- Place your feet flat on the floor and sit up straight in the chair.

- While you inhale, raise your arms in the air.

- Fold forward while exhaling, bringing the hands to the feet.

- Hold for a little while, then raise yourself back up to a sitting posture gradually.

Pose of the Half-Pigeon

- Sit up straight in the chair, flat on the floor.

- Gently lower the right knee toward the floor while crossing the right ankle across the left knee.

- Hold for a few seconds, then release, and repeat on the other side.

Standing Forward Bend

- Step forward while bending at the waist while keeping your toes pointed front.

- While you inhale, raise your arms in the air.

- Fold forward while exhaling, bringing the hands to the feet.

- Hold for a few while, then gently raise yourself back up to standing.

Wide Leg Forward Bend

- Standing with your feet apart and your toes pointed forward, do a wide-legged forward bend.

- While you inhale, raise your arms in the air.

- Fold forward while exhaling, bringing the hands to the floor in front of the feet.

- Hold for a few while, then gently raise yourself back up to standing.

Seniors who practice these hip openers and forward folds may improve their lower back and hip mobility, as well as relieve stress and pain.

Cool Down Pose

Every yoga practice, particularly chair yoga for seniors, must include cool-down postures. They ease stress and anxiety, aid in the body's recovery after exercise, and enhance general wellbeing. Here are some relaxation positions for elders to try:

Seated Forward Bend with a Twist

- Place your feet flat on the ground and sit up straight in the chair.
- While you inhale, raise your arms in the air.
- Fold forward while exhaling, bringing the hands to the feet.
- Then turn to the right, putting the right hand on the chair's back and the left hand on the right knee.

- Hold for a few seconds, then release, and repeat on the other side.

Sitting Spinal Twist

- Place your feet flat on the floor and sit up straight in the chair.
- Twisting to the right, place the right hand behind the back and the left hand on the right knee.
- Hold for a little while, then release, and repeat on the other side.

Child's Pose

- Kneel on the floor with the knees hip-width apart and the toes touching.
- Reach the arms forward and place the forehead on the floor, resting the arms alongside the body.
- Hold for a little while, then release.

Legs up the Wall Pose

- Lie on your back and lean sideways against a wall.

- Swing your legs up the wall.

- Breathe deeply while you rest your arms next to your body.

- Hold for a while, then gently bring the legs back to the starting position.

Corpse Pose

- Arms, legs, and palms up in the corpse position while you lay on your back.

- Focus on relaxing the whole body while you close your eyes and take deep breaths.

- Hold for a while, then raise your legs gradually.

Seniors may benefit from these relaxation and stress-relieving positions that also encourage tranquility and general wellbeing.

Chapter Four

Benefits of Chair Yoga for Seniors

A moderate variation of yoga that may be done while sitting or with a chair's support is called chair yoga. For seniors over 60 who may have restricted mobility, chronic pain, or other medical issues that make regular yoga positions challenging, it is an excellent form of exercise. The following are some advantages of chair yoga for seniors:

Age-related improvements in flexibility, strength, and balance may be achieved via chair yoga positions. Seniors may expand their range of motion, develop muscular strength, and enhance their general balance and coordination by doing mild stretches and postures. This may enhance general physical function and quality of life while also assisting in the prevention of falls and other mishaps.

Seniors who practice chair yoga may also see a decrease in tension and anxiety. Deep breathing exercises and relaxation methods may assist to settle the mind and encourage a feeling of relaxation and well-being. Seniors who may be struggling with chronic pain, disease, or other difficulties in their life may find this to be of particular use.

Improved joint mobility and pain management: Seniors who have joint discomfort or stiffness may find chair yoga to be beneficial. The mild exercises and stretches may ease discomfort and increase joint mobility, making it simpler for elders to move about and go about their regular tasks. The use of breathing exercises and relaxation methods may also lessen inflammation and enhance general pain management.

Improved mental clarity and concentration: Seniors who practice chair yoga might also benefit from improved mental clarity and attention. Seniors who utilize mindfulness and meditation practices may remain focused and present in the moment, which is particularly beneficial for those who may be experiencing memory loss or cognitive impairment.

Chair yoga may assist seniors in breathing and circulation improvement. Seniors may boost oxygen flow throughout their bodies and improve lung function by practicing deep breathing exercises. Seniors who may be struggling with breathing problems or other chronic diseases that impair breathing may find this to be very helpful.

Chair yoga is a risk-free and efficient type of exercise for seniors over 60 that may aid in enhancing breathing and circulation, reducing stress and anxiety, managing joint pain, and improving flexibility, strength, and balance. Prior to starting any new fitness regimen, including chair yoga, seniors should speak with their healthcare physician. They should also practice under the supervision of a certified teacher.

Chapter Five

Frequently Asked Questions about Chair Yoga for Seniors over 60

Can seniors with physical limitations practice chair yoga?

The practice of chair yoga is possible for seniors with physical limitations. In fact, seniors who may have restricted mobility, chronic pain, or other medical issues that make conventional yoga postures challenging might consider chair yoga as a form of exercise.

To accommodate each participant's unique requirements and skills, chair yoga may be modified. A chair may be used as a prop to make adjustments and changes that make the exercise secure and open to everyone. Seniors who have limited mobility, for instance, may do moderate stretches and exercises while sitting in the chair, while those who have more mobility can integrate standing postures while supported by the chair.

Instead of vigorous physical exercise, the emphasis of chair yoga is on soft motions, breath work, and relaxation methods. As a result, it is a risk-free and efficient type of exercise for seniors who may suffer from ailments like arthritis, osteoporosis, or persistent discomfort.

Seniors who have physical restrictions should speak with their doctor before starting any new fitness regimen, including chair yoga. It is also advised to practice under the supervision of a trained teacher who can make adjustments and provide help as needed.

Overall, chair yoga is a fantastic, safe, and easily accessible option for seniors with physical limitations to increase their flexibility, strength, balance, and general well-being.

How often need seniors to do chair yoga?

The frequency of senior chair yoga practice might vary based on the person's health, degree of fitness, and objectives. But as a general rule, older citizens should try to do chair yoga at least twice or three times every week.

Gaining the advantages of chair yoga requires consistency. Seniors' flexibility, strength, balance, and general health may all be improved with regular practice. Also, it's important to pay attention to the body and practice at a tempo that is both secure and comfortable.

The duration and intensity of their practice should be progressively increased over time for seniors who are new to chair yoga or have physical restrictions. They may choose to begin with shorter, more frequent practice sessions. To develop a practice regimen that is both secure and efficient, it is crucial to speak with a trained teacher and healthcare professional.

For their general health and well-being, seniors should practice chair yoga regularly in addition to engaging in other physical activities and good lifestyle practices like walking, stretching, strength training, and eating a balanced diet.

What times of day are ideal for doing chair yoga?

Depending on each person's schedule and preferences, there may be a different optimum time of day to practice chair yoga. However, there are other periods of the day when doing chair yoga could be better for elders.

It's common for elders to do yoga in the morning since it might give them a peaceful head start on the day. Seniors may benefit from chair yoga to enhance their circulation, wake up their body and mind, and establish a great mood for the remainder of the day.

The middle of the day might also be a good time for chair yoga since it can give seniors a break from prolonged sitting and increase their energy and attention. Seniors who include chair yoga into their midday routines report feeling more alert, having less stress and anxiety, and having better posture and breathing.

A wonderful time to practice chair yoga is in the evening since it may assist seniors unwind and unwind before bed. Seniors who practice chair yoga may relieve any tension or stress that has built up over the day, encourage relaxation and better sleep, and get the body and mind ready for a peaceful night's sleep.

Ultimately, the best time of day to practice chair yoga is when it fits into the individual's schedule and can be done consistently. Seniors should choose a time of day that works best for them and their lifestyle, whether it's early morning, mid-day, or evening, and make chair yoga a regular part of their routine.

What should seniors do if they are hurt or feel uncomfortable while practicing?

It's crucial to halt a posture or exercise if an elderly person feels pain or discomfort when practicing chair yoga and examine the situation. Pain or discomfort may indicate that a position or exercise is being performed improperly or that the body is not ready for it.

Seniors should pay attention to their bodies and avoid pushing themselves too far. They should always practice within their comfort range, and if they are hurting or uncomfortable, they should tell their teacher.

Seniors should speak with their healthcare professional if pain or discomfort continues so they can discover the underlying reason and whether chair yoga is still a good type of exercise for them. To account for physical restrictions or medical issues, changes or alternative postures could be required in certain situations.

Seniors should warm up adequately before practice and use breathing exercises to ease physical strain and stress. Seniors may customize their practice to fit their unique needs and skills with the assistance of a skilled teacher, who can also lead them through a secure and productive chair yoga session.

Chapter Six

Conclusion

For seniors over 60 who want to increase their flexibility, strength, balance, and general health, chair yoga is an excellent type of exercise. Chair yoga is suitable for seniors of all physical abilities and fitness levels because of its focus on slow, gentle movements and breath work.

There are a variety of advantages to chair yoga for seniors over 60, including increased breathing and circulation, less tension and anxiety, greater joint mobility, improved mental clarity, and pain management. These advantages may result in an improved quality of life, more freedom, and a feeling of general well-being.

We recommend giving chair yoga a go if you are a senior over 60 in order to lead a healthy lifestyle. You may reap the numerous advantages of this low-impact fitness program with consistent practice. Chair yoga may keep you active, healthy, and content as you age, whether you practice at home or in a group environment. Before beginning any new workout program, always get the advice of a trained teacher and healthcare professional.

www.ingramcontent.com/pod-product-compliance
Lightning Source LLC
Chambersburg PA
CBHW070804250726
48662CB00004B/1977